A CAREER AS A CARDIOVASCULAR TECHNOLOGIST

DO YOU ENJOY HELPING PEOPLE? Would you like to work with state-of-the-art technology? Are you interested in a profession in a skyrocketing segment of the allied healthcare field?

These attractive features and many more, characterize the burgeoning specialty of Cardiovascular Technology. Employment of CVTs is expected to increase by a whopping 25 percent within the next decade.

A trio of factors account for this career's upward trajectory, two of which are related to the aging population: the Baby Boom generation, 76 million strong, started turning 60 in 2007. People are living longer, thanks to continual advances in healthcare and medicine. The third factor is distressing: Americans, generally, do not take good care of their own health.

Heart disease is a phenomenon of the modern age. In pre-industrial societies, most people's livelihoods consisted of manual labor. Domestic life involved vigorous activity by men, women, and even children. Before people had access to manufactured products and the conveniences of modern life, they were largely self-sufficient. American pioneers cut down trees for firewood, built their own and their neighbors' houses, repaired their own roofs, hunted for food, drew water from the well, churned milk into butter, harvested crops, sheared sheep, slaughtered their own livestock, played stickball and hopscotch, and walked to school. Tobacco and sugar were luxuries for most people, who had little discretionary spending money and lived far from the general store, if there was one. Food was plentiful at harvest time, but scarce in the winter.

Today, our homes are heated and cooled with the flick of a switch. Water flows through our taps, our food comes from the supermarket, and high-tech entertainment devices have replaced physical activity as young people's recreation of choice. Those who are old enough to purchase them easily obtain tobacco and alcohol. Foods laden with sugar, salt and fat are readily available at chain restaurants, as prepared frozen meals, and right off the shelf in the form of chips and other savory snacks. We do not walk to the corner store anymore, because there is not one. Instead, we drive to the mall. If we want to exercise, we go to the gym. Nevertheless, mostly we sit on the couch in front of the TV or in a chair in front of the computer screen.

All of these dietary and lifestyle factors contribute to conditions implicated in heart disease, including high blood pressure, obesity, atherosclerosis (narrowing of the arteries that obstructs blood flow to the heart), and elevated levels of cholesterol, the soft, waxy substance that builds up in the blood, causing atherosclerosis. Hypercholesterolemia may sometimes be an inherited condition, but often it is related to excessive consumption of saturated fat and dietary cholesterol.

According to the American Heart Association, coronary heart disease is the leading cause of death in the United States, and stroke is the third leading cause of death.

Every year, 1.2 million Americans have a first or recurrent coronary attack, and more than 450,000 of these people die.

700,000 people suffer a new or recurrent stroke and more than 150,000 of them die.

Nearly eight million adult Americans have survived a heart attack.

Nine million have angina pectoris, chest pain or discomfort caused by an insufficient supply of blood to the heart muscle.

An estimated 72 million adults have high blood pressure.

46 million men and women smoke cigarettes.

37 million adult Americans have cholesterol levels high enough to put them in considerable danger of developing coronary heart disease or suffering a stroke.

70 percent of Americans do not get adequate exercise.

Two-thirds of American adults are overweight.

Two-thirds of diabetics die from a cardiovascular-related disease.

What can a cardiovascular technologist do to help alleviate these terrible healthcare problems?

Working under the direction of a cardiologist (heart specialist) or other medical doctor, the CVT performs procedures on patients that are used in the diagnosis and treatment of cardiac (heart) and peripheral vascular (blood vessel) diseases. Data are collected from these procedures and interpreted by the doctor to determine the presence and degree of heart disease.

Other duties may include reviewing and recording patients' medical histories, scheduling appointments, and recording into a database the physician's assessments of the diagnostic findings.

Cardiovascular technologists usually choose one of these specialties: Invasive Cardiology, Noninvasive Cardiology or Noninvasive Vascular Technology.

In the cardiac procedures termed "invasive," the medical team enters the patient's body in order to insert the catheter tubing, which may be equipped with devices like angioplasty balloons or rotating shavers; to insert cardiac stents; to implant pacemakers; and to perform open-heart surgery.

Noninvasive medical technology refers to safe, painless procedures that are performed outside the patient's body. Perhaps the best-known noninvasive procedure is diagnostic medical sonography (DMS), an imaging technique that uses ultrasound, or high-frequency sound waves, to view the internal structure and function of the human body. You are probably familiar with the use of sonograms during pregnancy to monitor the health and growth of a fetus (obstetric sonography). The various job titles of ultrasound specialists in the cardiovascular field include Cardiac Sonographer, Cardiovascular Sonographer, Echocardiographer, Vascular Technologist, and Vascular Sonographer.

Intrigued? This report tells you all about exploring and preparing for a job in cardiovascular technology, what kind of education is required, what you will earn, benefits and drawbacks to this work, and everything else you need to know about a career centered on that magnificent muscle, the heart!

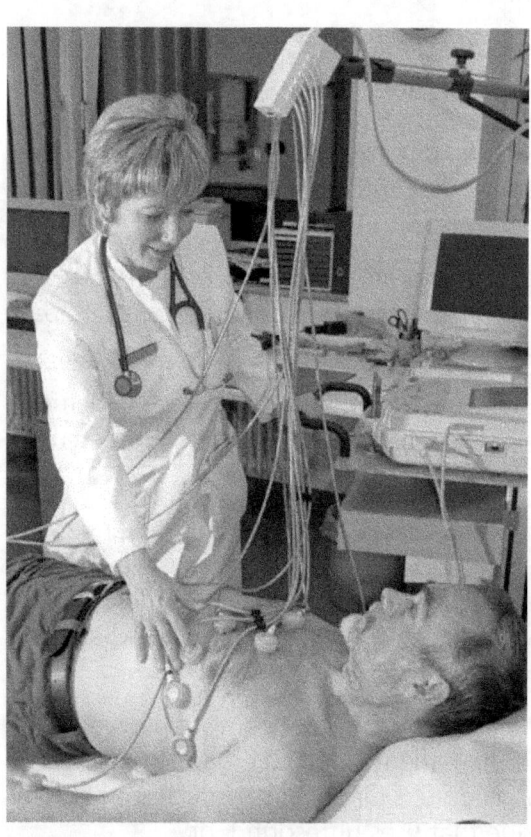

THINGS TO DO NOW

Schooling

There are many ways to explore this career that will help you determine whether you have the interest, skills, and temperament necessary to become a cardiovascular technologist.

One of the most important things you can do now is assess your academic aptitude for math and science. Take as many classes as your high school offers in math (algebra and calculus), biology, chemistry, anatomy and physiology, and physics. Because CVTs interact constantly with other members of the medical team as well as with patients, public speaking, communications, psychology, and sociology are often part of a professional program's core curriculum. It is important that you enjoy studying these subjects, as your professional education will continue throughout your career.

Do you have to enroll in a professional training program? In short, yes. Although CVTs in the past have often received on-the-job training, the growing status and professionalism that characterize this occupation call for a more formal educational approach. With an Associate of Science or Associate of Applied Science degree, your employment prospects and opportunities for career advancement will be much stronger. Indeed, there is a growing trend that has healthcare facilities and insurance companies requiring degrees and professional credentials of job applicants.

Instruction is offered at community colleges, junior colleges, vocational and technical schools, universities, hospitals, and medical schools. Four-year college programs that provide training for future CVTs are also emerging. While the advantages of earning a bachelor's degree are many, two-year programs are considerably more affordable and graduates are qualified for most entry-level jobs.

It is essential that you choose a program that is accredited by the Commission on Accreditation of Allied Health Education Programs, listed at http://www.caahep.org/Find-An-Accredited-Program. Accreditation means that the program's curricula, policies and procedures meet a set of standards and guidelines developed by the Joint Review Committee on Education in Cardiovascular Technology. Now is a good time to start exploring the various programs. The CAAHEP website allows you to search by profession (look under Cardiovascular Technologist or Diagnostic Medical Sonographer); by concentration (for CVT, they include Cardiac Electrophysiology, Invasive Cardiology, Noninvasive Cardiology, and Noninvasive Peripheral Vascular); by state; by accreditation status; by degree/credential (diploma, certificate, associate or bachelor's).

About 35 CVT and 170 DMS programs have been awarded accreditation. Research several programs to get a feel for what the education is like. Does the curriculum intrigue you? Are you excited by the prospect of being in the lab, interacting with the faculty, completing internships?

Technical Ability

You probably already know whether you have the flair for technology and mechanics that CVTs need in order to utilize the sophisticated equipment and precise instruments integral to their work. Do you enjoy working on a computer? Do you learn how to use new software and applications readily? Are you comfortable and confident in your science lab classes?

Learn More

Consider enrolling in a cardiopulmonary resuscitation (CPR) course to see if you're comfortable with the physical contact CVTs have with their patients. Even if your "patient" is a dummy, the experience will be enlightening. CPR is a skill cardiovascular technologists need and everyone else should possess as well! You can find a local class through the American Heart Association at this website: http://www.americanheart.org/presenter.jhtml ?identifier=3012360.

By volunteering at a hospital, you can decide whether you enjoy working in a healthcare setting. You will not have direct contact with patients in any medical context, but you will have the opportunity to ask practicing CVTs about the profession.

See if your biology teacher can obtain an educational video of a real-life angioplasty or coronary artery surgery to show the class. (You can also find short videos on YouTube.) Many CVTs who initially chose other occupations say they were "hooked" or "sold" on the career when they observed their first cardiac procedure.

HISTORY OF THIS CAREER

GREAT STRIDES WERE MADE IN THE field of cardiology from the 17th century to the early 20th century, including the inventions of the stethoscope and the electrocardiograph, the first descriptions of the circulatory system and the anatomical structure of the heart, and the first instances of blood pressure measurement, catheterization, cardiac surgery, and the use of defibrillation to restore the heartbeat to normal.

It was not until 1912 that trailblazing cardiologist Dr. James B. Herrick first articulated a clinical definition of heart disease. The American Heart Association, whose Council on Clinical Cardiology presents an annual James B. Herrick Award to a physician who has made profound contributions to advancement and practice in the field, describes Dr. Herrick as a pioneer. "His contributions were many, but perhaps most significant was his classic paper," states the AHA. "Besides giving the medical world a definitive description of coronary thrombosis, his studies emphasized the important observation that sudden obstruction of a coronary artery is not necessarily fatal."

That classic paper, titled Clinical Features of Sudden Obstruction of the Coronary Arteries was presented to members of the Association of American Physicians in 1912. The prevailing theory at the time was that myocardial infarction (heart attack) inevitably caused sudden death because coronary arteries were not connected to any other blood vessels. Dr. Herrick argued a myocardial infarction was not necessarily fatal; full recovery is possible. He posited there could be a number of contributing factors in a heart attack unrelated to the arterial system's ending at the heart. Among them are whether the membrane that surrounds the heart is inflamed and irritated, the condition of the undamaged parts of the heart, and the presence of cardiogenic shock. (Weak pulse, low blood pressure, clammy skin, bulging jugular veins, hyperventilation, and other signs may characterize this condition.)

Dr. Herrick's presentation landed with a thud, but his reputation was ensured in 1918 with his seminal paper that definitively described coronary thrombosis (a blood clot creating blockage in the arteries). The following decades saw the first recorded human cardiac catheterization using X-ray techniques, and the first use of the cardiac catheter as a diagnostic tool to investigate cardiac function.

Since World War II, technological advances in treatments for cardiovascular diseases have accelerated. Milestones have been achieved and surpassed in antibiotics, anesthesia, blood transfusions, sonography, open-heart surgery, heart-lung machines, coronary angiography, heart transplantation, angioplasty, coronary stents, rotational atherectomy devices, and intravascular ultrasound.

As cardiovascular diseases reached epidemic proportions, the need for healthcare providers trained in this field became more urgent. As equipment and devices developed to diagnose and treat heart ailments grew more sophisticated, the need for technicians with specialized knowledge and training intensified.

In 1981, the American Medical Association granted Cardiovascular Technology official status as an allied health profession. Standards for the accreditation of CVT education programs were established in 1983. The Joint Review Committee on Education in Cardiovascular Technology convened for the first time in 1985. Three years later, Cardiovascular Credentialing International was established in 1988.

Credentialing organizations already existed at the time – the

American Registry for Diagnostic Medical Sonography was incorporated in 1975, but registry/certification has become increasingly critical for all parties.

For the CVT profession, credentialing enhances its reputation and credibility. Employers prefer credentialed employees because they have already demonstrated their knowledge, ability, and commitment by passing the exams. If the CVT is certified in more than one specialty, that employee is even more valuable. Insurance companies want healthcare facilities to hire credentialed professionals to protect them against liability.

CVT organizations continually strive to standardize academic and professional requirements, further enhancing the credibility and respect afforded this profession and its practitioners. In 2007, Cardiovascular Credentialing International began administering the Registered Cardiac Electrophysiology Specialist designation.

In 2008, the Society of Diagnostic Medical Sonography announced that a consensus of 18 medical organizations had produced a curriculum guideline for sonography education and training.

WHERE YOU WILL WORK

THERE ARE ALMOST 50,000 CARDIOVASCULAR technologists and technicians employed in the United States. About three in four are employed by public and private general medical and surgical hospitals. Invasive cardiovascular technologists may work in operating rooms or open-heart surgical suites.

Another 15 percent work in physicians' offices.

Four percent of cardiovascular technologists and technicians are employed by outpatient care centers, medical and diagnostic laboratories, and providers of ambulatory healthcare services, such as imaging and pacemaker monitoring. Employees of mobile diagnostic, surgical, and healthcare clinics travel from site to site, wherever the patients they serve are located.

Various types of labs employ CVTs. Those specializing in invasive medicine work in cardiac catheterization and electrophysiology labs. Noninvasive cardiovascular technologists are likely found in echocardiography, stress test, and electrocardiography labs. Vascular CVTs are employed in laboratories equipped with an array of sonographic technology.

A small number of CVTs are educators in junior colleges, four-year colleges and universities, and professional schools. CVTs also find jobs with cardiac rehabilitation centers, cardiac research facilities, extended care facilities, emergency clinics, public health facilities, and health maintenance organizations (HMOs). Some work in sales or marketing in private industry, where salaries are higher and opportunities for advancement are more plentiful.

The number of CVTs working in certain employment settings is expected to show tremendous growth in the coming decade. For example, the number of CVTs working in hospitals is expected to increase by over 20 percent. Similarly, the number of cardiovascular technologists and technicians employed by mobile healthcare providers will soar by over 50 percent. Employment growth in these other employer categories is expected to be especially strong:

Specialty hospitals

Offices of health practitioners other than doctors

Ambulance services

Administrative and support services

Physicians' offices

Outpatient care centers

Medical and diagnostic laboratories

Geographically, cardiovascular technologists are located wherever healthcare facilities are. CVTs whose jobs require them to be "on call" for emergencies are expected to live within 30 minutes of their employers.

THE WORK YOU WILL DO

Invasive Cardiovascular Technologist

The primary role of the invasive CVT is to assist and support the cardiologist or cardiac surgeon in performing cardiac catheterizations, a procedure that is also known as an angiogram. To perform this procedure, a physician, assisted by cardiovascular technicians, inserts a long, thin, flexible tube, called a catheter, into a blood vessel in the patient's leg, arm, groin, or neck. Guided by X-ray pictures projected on a monitor, the physician threads the catheter into the coronary arteries. A special dye is injected through the catheter, illuminating the heart and arteries on the X-ray machine.

Cardiac catheterization helps the physician determine whether there is a blockage or narrowing in the blood vessels that supply the heart muscle, which coronary arteries are affected, and how severely. The procedure also helps the physician assess the overall functioning of the heart muscle and valves, the extent of the damage after a heart attack, and the next steps in treatment.

During the procedure, the patient is given a mild sedative to promote relaxation but remains awake to allow any necessary communication between patient and doctor to take place. The test takes about an hour and usually does not cause the patient discomfort, with the exception of some soreness at the insertion site and grogginess from the sedative. Complications from the procedure are rare.

Based on what the angiogram finds, the physician may recommend balloon angioplasty. In this procedure, a tiny balloon is affixed to the end of the catheter. When the instrument reaches the site of the coronary artery in question, the balloon is inflated and the buildup of obstructive plaque is forced against the artery walls. Balloon angioplasty is used to treat blockages of blood vessels or heart valves and to restore blood flow.

In seven out of 10 cases, a small, collapsible, mesh tube called a coronary stent is used during an angioplasty. The stent is attached to the catheter and installed at the site of the blockage, where it self-expands and forms a kind of scaffold that holds the artery open. It is left there permanently, and a few weeks after the procedure the tissue that lines the artery begins to grow over the surface of the device.

Another catheter-based procedure that serves essentially the same purposes as an angioplasty is atherectomy, in which a rotating shaver, a sharp blade, or lasers are attached to the end of the tube and used to slice away or vaporize the plaque.

CVTs participate in every step of the catheterization procedure. Beforehand, they tell the patient all about what to expect, answer any questions, secure a signed informed consent form, set up the sterile field, arrange the X-ray equipment that is used to guide the catheter up into the heart, and make sure that life-saving measures are at the ready. A CVT positions the patient on an examining table, shaves and cleans the small portion of the body where the catheter will be inserted, and applies an anesthetic to this area.

The members of the CVT team usually include scrub assistant, monitoring assistant, and circulating assistant. Scrub assistants scrub in themselves, and then prep and drape the patient. They then assist the physician with the instruments and medications required during the procedure.

The monitoring CVT keeps track of the patient's vital signs with EKG equipment, operating the computerized recording system and maintaining documentation of the procedure. The patient's hemodynamics (derived from the words for blood and motion, hemodynamics describes blood flow/circulation) are monitored, and a special sensor is used to observe vein and artery pressure within the heart. Monitoring CVTs inform the physician if something appears to be wrong or troubling. Monitors also perform the calculations used by the physician to determine whether a patient has to be admitted for open-heart surgery.

Circulatory CVTs are mobile during the procedure, attending to the needs of the patient and administering the medications. They are also responsible for handing equipment to the physician and scrub assistant as needed.

Some invasive CVTs prep and monitor patients undergoing open-heart surgery and operations for the implantation of pacemakers. They may also administer clot-dissolving drugs, operate mechanical devices known as cardiac assist pumps for patients with pacemakers, and support other cardiac emergency procedures.

Noninvasive Cardiovascular Technologist

Noninvasive CVTs are involved primarily with performing examinations, recording and analyzing data, and submitting findings to the physician for interpretation. The technology and equipment typically used in noninvasive cardiovascular laboratories include transesophageal and stress echocardiograms; electrocardiograms (EKG or ECG); Holter monitoring; and pacemaker monitoring and reprogramming.

Echocardiograms use ultrasound, or high-frequency sound waves, to generate images of the internal structures of the heart, enabling the physician to evaluate how well the heart is working based on the size of the chambers, how well the valves are working, how well the pumping ventricles are functioning, and whether there are structural defects present. Echocardiograms provide more detail and are safer than X-rays. CVTs who use ultrasound are known as cardiac sonographers or echocardiographers.

In echocardiography, the CVT applies gel and electrodes to the patient's chest and passes a probe known as a transducer over the chest area to produce images from various angles. The test takes between one-half hour and 90 minutes.

In a transesophageal echocardiogram (TEE), the transducer is fed by the CVT through the mouth and throat into the esophagus and positioned behind the heart to collect the ultrasound images. This procedure is slightly more risky than a conventional echocardiogram mainly because of the possibility that the procedure might cause the patient to gag.

Electrocardiograph (EKG) cardiovascular technicians administer electrocardiograms, which record the electrical impulses produced by the beating heart. To accomplish this, electrodes are attached to the patient's chest, arms, and legs. The atria and ventricles produce waves that represent the electrical impulses as they travel to the upper and lower chambers. It also measures activity when the ventricles are in a resting state.

The CVT makes a printout of the reading on EKG graph paper that can then be interpreted by the physician. The information helps the doctor determine whether the heartbeat's electrical activity is normal, slow, fast, or irregular; what part of the heart was damaged if a heart attack had occurred; whether there is a sufficient supply of blood and oxygen to the heart; and whether the patient has an enlarged heart, which signifies heart disease. Electrocardiography is performed prior to surgery and is part of a routine physical exam among older and at-risk patients.

EKGs are safe and painless and take no longer than 10 minutes.

Specially trained EKG technicians are qualified to administer Holter monitor and exercise stress testing. In the former, electrodes are placed on the patient's chest and a portable or ambulatory EKG monitor is strapped to the patient's waist or belt, a fairly complicated process that takes about 15 minutes. The patient resumes normal activity for 24 hours while the device records the electrical activity of the heart. After this period, the technician scans the recording tape onto an electronic screen, checks the quality of the data, and prints the results for later interpretation by the physician. The data are used to diagnose such ailments as arrhythmias (heartbeat abnormalities) and problems with pacemakers.

Exercise stress tests (also known as stress tests, exercise tolerance tests, exercise EKGs, or treadmill tests) document the heart's electrical activity during exertion. The patient is connected with electrodes to the EKG monitor. Baseline readings of cardiac activity and resting blood pressure are recorded. Next, the patient walks on a motorized treadmill, with the speed gradually being accelerated, while the technician observes the effect of increasingly vigorous exercise on the heart's performance. The patient may be on the treadmill for as long as 15 minutes, but the test is halted if the patient experiences discomfort.

In a nuclear stress test, the CVT injects dyes into the bloodstream to provide even more information about the blood flow to the heart.

Changes in the EKG pattern and symptoms the patient has experienced help the doctor evaluate such cardiac conditions as arrhythmia, the impact exercise has on the blood and oxygen flow to the heart, recovery speed, the patient's degree of cardiovascular conditioning, and target heart rate for cardiovascular exercise.

Vascular Technologists

Those CVTs known as vascular technologists or vascular sonographers also use noninvasive techniques, notably ultrasound. They specialize in the vascular, or circulatory system, which is made up of blood vessels (arteries, veins, and capillaries). A related area of expertise is the cerebrovascular system, pertaining to the delivery of blood to the brain. This is of concern because damage or a blockage in one of these arteries can lead to a stroke, which has sometimes been referred to as a "heart attack of the brain." In fact, stroke is frequently caused by a blood clot that travels through the bloodstream from the heart to the brain.

After recording the patient's medical history, explaining the procedure, and responding to questions and concerns, VTs proceed with the examination.

VTs are especially skilled at using a combination of qualitative (observation and interpretation) and quantitative (data collection) techniques to perform their diagnostic procedures. When conducting the scan, VTs scrutinize images to distinguish between healthy and diseased tissue, use their judgment to select images for evaluation, and determine whether the visual documentation is sufficient for a diagnosis. They then summarize their findings for submission to the physician.

The VT may also use ultrasound to record blood volume, blood pressure, and blood flow in the patient's legs. The legs are examined to check for peripheral artery disease, in which "peripheral" blood vessels (those outside the heart and brain) are narrowed by the buildup of fatty deposits. Peripheral artery disease is the most common type of peripheral vascular disease, and it can lead to gangrene and amputation, and, if the debris travels to the cerebrovascular system, heart attack and stroke. Morbidity rates are high. Yet many of those afflicted do not realize anything is wrong because symptoms are mild at first: some discomfort while walking, which people may just associate with aging, and slight discoloration of the feet.

Advancement

CVTs who advance to supervisory positions assume more managerial and administrative duties, such as:

Coordinating day-to-day operations of the catheterization lab (usually called the "cath lab")

Supervising the maintenance of ultrasound equipment and recommending upgrades

Preparing schedules in cooperation with the charge nurse to ensure smooth patient flow

Ensuring that the technical and procedural standards of the lab meet professional and regulatory requirements

Ordering supplies, negotiating with vendors, and remaining within the department budget

Training, mentoring, and evaluating staff

Some CVTs may move into other, related occupations, such as medical equipment sales or teaching.

CARDIOVASCULAR TECHNOLOGISTS TALK ABOUT THEIR CAREERS

I Am the Director of Cardiovascular and Pulmonary Services for a Medical Center in North Carolina

"I began my career in the cardiovascular world in the military. When I read the training they offered and the description duties I would have, I was intrigued. I felt it would be a way to stretch and promote my military career. After the training and as I began to acquire some expertise in the field I realized that the cardiovascular field was much more exciting than my military career. So I decided to leave the Army and pursue a career at a hospital that would challenge me with complex interventions and research. I chose Carolinas Medical Center in Charlotte, North Carolina. I am credentialed as a Registered Cardiovascular Invasive Specialist and a Registered Cardiac Electrophysiology Specialist. I also have a BS degree in Health Administration.

My current position is purely administrative. My prior position was Technical Supervisor of the Cardiac Cath Lab at Carolinas Medical Center, and I served in this capacity for 10 years. I was responsible negotiating contracts with vendors, accessing new technology, managing the computer networks within the labs, physician liaison, employee supervision, and capital project supervision. I also was able to work in the labs as needed, such as when we were short-staffed.

The first and most important thing you need to do when starting your career is to listen. Most experienced technologists would love to pass on the knowledge and insights they have acquired over the years.

The most important thing you can do to advance your career

is to take as much on-call duty as possible. Not only do you get to see and learn how to handle the sickest of patients, which provides invaluable experience and training, but also the physicians get to know you and to trust your judgment. Nothing gives you a greater sense of accomplishment than a seasoned cardiologist asking your opinion of the best treatment for their patient! ("What do you think, 3.0 or 3.5 stent?")

When you go on job interviews, dress the part of a professional. You are interviewing for a career, not a job bagging groceries. Men, put on a conservative jacket and tie; women should be in business suit or dress. I have had people come in shorts and flip-flops and I do not even waste my time on them.

Ask questions during the interview. Show them you are engaged and interested in the types of procedures, the physicians' groups that practice in the lab, and the opportunities for advancement.

Join a professional organization. I would be sure to join the Society of Invasive Cardiovascular Professionals, for example."

I Started as a Firefighter and Paramedic

"Prior to working in this field, I had been working as a paramedic and firefighter. I enjoyed taking care of acutely injured and sick patients, but after many years I had become tired of dealing with many patients who weren't in that bad condition. A firefighter's schedule allows for part-time employment and I was always very interested in working with heart patients, which led me to apply for a part-time position at our local hospital.

I initially started as a noninvasive cardiovascular technician performing 12-lead ECGs and assisting with exercise treadmill tests. I spent every spare minute when not doing ECGs and treadmills in the cardiac cath lab observing cases. I was very impressed with the degree of knowledge of the cardiovascular technologists, and this motivated me to learn more. I was fascinated with the technology utilized and procedures performed in the cath lab that helped patients so tremendously.

Today, I serve as Director for Cardiology and Endoscopy Services at a medical center in Ogden, Utah. There were no cardiovascular programs in the state where I live, but I was able to find a distance learning program that I could participate in. That's where I eventually graduated from. I will admit that my experience and education as a paramedic was very helpful to me, but that background would not be a prerequisite to pursuing this career. There are many great educational programs across the US, and I would recommend this route if it is available to you. I know that in some areas that lack a program in the vicinity, it is not uncommon to find on-the-job training as a pathway into this profession.

Obtaining the Registered Cardiovascular Invasive Specialist (RCIS) credential is encouraged because employers are looking for credentialed, competent cardiovascular technologists. This credential requires passing an exam to demonstrate fundamental competency, and continuing education to maintain the credential.

For me, the greatest reward comes when you have a critically ill patient in the middle of a heart attack, and then you see immediate relief when a blocked coronary artery is opened. It's an awesome feeling! I also really enjoy working in an environment where you work closely as a team taking care of patients. Personally, I really enjoy taking care of the very sick patient. Perhaps it stems from my days as a paramedic!

I would highly recommend that you take any medically related courses such as medical terminology, human biology, emergency medical services, certified nurse's aide/assistant training, and chemistry. These will all create a great background for someone interested in the field of cardiovascular science."

I Am a Registered Cardiovascular Invasive Specialist Employed in a Cardiac Catheterization Lab

"I was working as an EMT in an emergency department and had a patient that was having an inferior myocardial infarction. We brought the patient to the cardiovascular lab and I was able to stay and observe the procedure. I was hooked. This patient was diaphoretic, hypotensive, vomiting, and had severe chest pain when triaged. One hour and forty five minutes after we brought her in, she left the cath lab pain free with an open right coronary artery that had been totally occluded. I knew I had found my true calling.

Clinically, my responsibilities today are as follows:

Scrub on diagnostic and interventional cardiac catheterizations as well as permanent pacemaker and intra cardiac defibrillators.

Monitor patient's hemodynamics pre, during, and post procedure.

Circulate and run various equipment used to diagnose and treat coronary artery disease.

I am also in charge of managing the inventory in the department, handling the staff yearly competencies, and performing educational presentations for other staff in our facility and outside the hospital, such as at radiology schools.

In addition, I serve as Advocacy Committee Chair for the

Society of Invasive Cardiovascular Professionals.

Some of the qualities a cardiovascular technologist should have are a strong interest in science and an enjoyment of learning new things, because technology in the cardiovascular field is forever changing. Hours are long, and the work is both physically and mentally demanding, but I can't think of a more rewarding job.

Consider your schooling from day one – you need to be motivated, flexible, consistent, and personable."

I Have Over 25 Years of Experience as a Sonographer

"I was always interested in the medical field, and ultrasound incorporated many of my specific interests. Fields addressing the anatomy and physiology of the human body are always changing because of improvements in the technology. The ultrasound world is very rewarding because the patient's life can change with what you see inside that person.

I am doing all the different ultrasound specialties – abdominal, obstetrical, gynecological, and vascular, so I can examine a pregnant patient looking at the fetus, and the next patient can be a cancer patient or a patient with vascular problems. The different problems that those patients bring in front of me are the challenges of my working life. If the work I do can change a life for the better, I think my work is worthwhile. This is why I love my work.

Anyone who is doing any kind of ultrasound needs to be curious and have the desire to find an answer to a problem. You must be very observant to focus on and accurately read the images in front of you. You need to be very meticulous and disciplined, and to be versatile, because you are constantly dealing with people.

The rewards are worth all the effort. If you are looking for a very challenging profession, go for it! The demand is there, and growing. We need intelligent and dedicated people to take up the challenge."

PERSONAL QUALIFICATIONS

CVTS MUST HAVE TECHNICAL AND mechanical savvy. You will be working with highly sophisticated instruments and equipment on a daily basis. The patient will be comfortable with procedural steps – having electrodes attached to the body, for example – only if the technologist seems comfortable and confident. Healthcare facilities upgrade their equipment and introduce new technologies to remain state-of-the-art and provide the best possible care. Just as in the 1980s CVTs had to learn, alongside doctors, how angioplasties are performed, and in the 1990s they had to learn how to place stents, you must become skilled at using newly developed devices and machinery, and performing new procedures throughout your career.

Good manual dexterity and hand-eye coordination are also required, as are attention to detail and record-keeping skills.

Like all healthcare providers, cardiovascular technologists have top-notch interpersonal and communications skills. Explaining a technical procedure to a patient who may have little understanding of a health condition requires the CVT to communicate clearly, reassuringly, often using charts or anatomical models, without stumbling into abbreviations or medical jargon, and without condescending to the patient.

When engaging in physical contact with the patient, CVTs behave in a courteous, respectful manner and exhibit caring yet dispassionate confidence in their capabilities. To put anxious or frightened patients at ease when discussing impending procedures, diagnostic results and recommended therapies, cardiovascular technologists are both straightforward and tactful.

CVTs strike a delicate balance between patience and efficiency when it comes to answering patients' questions. This requires excellent listening skills. Is the patient interrogating you about the use of ultrasound or electrodes really wondering, "Am I going to die during this test?" Is a query like, "My brother-in-law had four open-heart surgeries and I'm wondering if that is normal," from someone who is about to undergo a routine stress test really an attempt to delay or avoid another lecture about smoking? Some patients may be skeptical about their rights of confidentiality. CVTs must address patients' concerns, while keeping in mind the necessity of performing the scheduled procedure and administering to the patients in the waiting room in a timely fashion.

Patients may feel so safe with a personable, calm CVT, that they may reveal information they have not told to their doctors. Conversely, cardiovascular technologists must behave in a professional manner if a patient seeks information that the CVT is not qualified or permitted to disclose. The patient will be advised to ask the question directly of the physician.

Communications and interpersonal skills are also necessary when actively functioning as a member of a medical team during a procedure. CVTs must respond immediately to a doctor's or a colleague's request and implement it without hesitation. In this capacity, teamwork and the ability to follow directions are critical.

Excellent judgment and analytical skills are required of CVTs, who are responsible for evaluating the findings of a diagnostic test and presenting them in a useful fashion to the physician. Cardiovascular technicians also need to alert the doctor if any worrisome signs are present, and they often work side-by-side with physicians in interpreting data.

To form solid judgments, to manage the stress inherent in a caregiving occupation, and to express kindness and forbearance when dealing with distraught patients and their families, cardiovascular technologists must be emotionally stable. Part of maintaining equilibrium is knowing how to take care of yourself, to blow off steam in a constructive way (biking, gardening, practicing martial arts, singing karaoke, taking a bubble bath, sleeping in).

CVTs in many occupations are required to meet physical requirements: the ability to hear commands uttered through surgical masks, to see equipment monitors from a distance, and to lift and transport both patients and diagnostic equipment.

ATTRACTIVE FEATURES

PRACTICING CARDIOVASCULAR TECHNOLOGISTS cite their service to patients as one of the greatest rewards of this career. One Registered Cardiovascular Invasive Specialist describes watching an obstructed blood vessel clear during an angioplasty as "an awesome feeling." Satisfaction with a job well done is familiar to everyone who is committed to a task. If you are a cardiovascular technologist, your well-done job may have helped save a life.

CVTs derive pleasure from their ability to educate cardiac patients one-on-one about their condition as well as their prevention and treatment options. CVTs not only assist in the diagnosis and treatment of serious cardiovascular conditions, they also enhance patients' knowledge of heart function, provide comfort, and promote peace of mind. It is a tremendous responsibility and honor to contribute directly to improving health and saving lives.

Another enjoyable interpersonal aspect of this career is the camaraderie among colleagues, especially those who work together in a cath lab. Working together under intense conditions as a team with a common purpose, supporting each other's efforts, exchanging roles as scrub assistant, monitoring assistant, and circulating assistant from one procedure to the next creates a powerful, almost familial bond.

No two days are the same in the professional life of a cardiovascular technologist. Every patient is different from every other, with an individual genetic makeup, medical history, lifestyle, and philosophical approach to health and healthcare. Each scan and catheterization reveals information that is one of a kind, every medical case is unique. Says one invasive cardiovascular technologist, "You're always dealing with someone new, and it's great just to meet all these different people. You are challenged by the different pathologies you see. It's something that you can do for a lifetime and never get bored, that's for sure!"

Medical technology is another ever-changing facet of this career. New drugs, devices, and equipment are always emerging. This is a boon to both patients and CVTs. The patient may be subjected to simpler and less invasive diagnostic procedures, benefit from earlier detection of diseases and other heart complications, and undergo treatments that are more effective and result in less discomfort. The cardiovascular technologist benefits from being able to provide better care, and enjoys the exciting and career-boosting challenge of learning to use new detection, diagnostic and treatment tools. CVTs evolve with the technology.

Employment opportunities for CVTs are excellent and will only become more so! The field of cardiovascular care is booming, due largely to the aging of the population. The risk of heart attack and strokes becomes significantly higher with age; and the percentage of the US population age 65 and older is expected to expand to over 20 percent by 2030. Accordingly, the number of employed cardiovascular technologists is expected to vault from about 45,000 currently to more than 60,000 in the near future.

UNATTRACTIVE FEATURES

NO QUESTION ABOUT IT, CARDIOVASCULAR technologists often work under stressful conditions. They regularly interact with people who have, or may have, serious heart disorders. Witnessing human suffering takes an emotional toll on all healthcare providers.

Procedures that rely on teamwork do not always progress with the efficiency of well-oiled machines. Medical teams are made up of human beings, who, regardless of their training and good intentions, are fallible. If a complication arises during catheterization or surgery, CVTs may find themselves unexpectedly facing a life-or-death situation.

CVTs have to strike a delicate balance between their professional and private lives: giving 110 percent when they are at work and then leaving the stress and distress behind when they go home.

The physical demands of the job can also take a toll. CVTs spend many hours standing, walking, lifting and turning patients and moving equipment. In addition, they may frequently perform repetitive tasks, and stand or sit in awkward positions during diagnostic testing. This can lead to musculoskeletal disorders including tendonitis, bursitis, pinched nerves in the wrist and neck, and back pain. Sonographers are in special risk because of the wrist posture required to use the transducer while twisting the head to watch the monitor. When you are a CVT, make sure your workspace is ergonomic.

Cardiovascular technologists are sometimes exposed to hazardous agents like acids, medical waste, anesthetic gases, infected blood, and radiation. This does not have to be an occupational hazard if you take the necessary precautions.

Sometimes CVTs are on emergency call during the night and on weekends, which can be disruptive to personal life and plans for rest, relaxation, and recreation.

EDUCATION AND TRAINING

CURRENTLY, THERE ARE 35 ACCREDITED education programs culminating in a diploma, certificate, associate degree, or bachelor's degree in cardiovascular technology. In addition, there are 168 accredited Diagnostic Medical Sonography programs. When researching the DMS programs, remember that they may specialize in cardiac, vascular, or general ultrasound diagnostics, so make sure you choose one with instruction and training aligned with your professional interests and goals.

Sampling of Associate Degree Programs

At this website you can search for schools offering associate degrees,

which generally require about two years to complete:
www.universities.com/edu/Associate_degrees_in_Cardiovascular
_Technology_Technologist.html

Here are descriptions of the programs at three different schools.

The Cardiovascular Technology program at Augusta Technical College in Georgia is offered in collaboration with the University Hospital's School of Cardiac and Vascular Technology. There are required courses as well as electives, including:

Abdominal Vascular

Advanced Cerebrovascular

Arterial Duplex

Basic Cerebrovascular and Venous Extremity

Basic Extremity Testing

Cardiac Cath Clinical

Cardiovascular Physiology

Cross Section Anatomy

Echocardiography Clinical

Electrophysiology

Essentials of Vascular Sonography

Interventional Therapeutic

Invasive Cardiovascular Fundamentals

Medical Physics

Noninvasive Cardiovascular Fundamentals

Sonography

Vascular Clinical

Vascular Physical Principles and Instrumentation

In addition to technical courses, students study the liberal arts (literature, psychology, history, math, science, and economics). www.augustatech.edu/AlliedHealth/degreeCardiovascular.shtml

The School of Allied Health at BryanLGH College of Health Sciences in Lincoln, Nebraska partners with BryanLGH Medical Center. The school offers the Associate of Science degree in Invasive Cardiovascular Technology, Associate of Science degree in Adult Cardiac Sonography, and Associate of Science degree in Vascular Sonography.

BryanLGH College of Health Sciences utilizes hands-on, adult and pediatric simulators designed to help students to apply their classroom learning to such tasks as administration of medication, infusion of intravenous fluid, and oxygen application.

http://dev.bryanlghcollege.org/go/academic-programs/school -of-allied-health

The Allied Health Department at Washington State's Spokane Community College offers two-year degree programs in the following specialties:

Invasive Cardiovascular Technology

Noninvasive Cardiovascular Technology

Diagnostic Medical Sonography

Vascular Technology

Students enrolled in the invasive and noninvasive cardiovascular programs spend three academic quarters together studying the core curriculum, which is designed to develop scientific, medical, and technical skills. In the second portion of the program, students in the invasive segment focus on cardiac catheterization and work in hospital cardiac labs in the Spokane area. Those studying noninvasive concentrate on the different methods of echocardiography. All students complete one academic quarter of internship at a major medical center outside the Spokane area.

http://www.scc.spokane.edu/?alliedh

Credentials

Once students have completed an accredited education program, they are eligible to sit for national certification and registry examinations administered by Cardiovascular Credentialing International (CCI) (www.cci-online.org) or the American Registry of Diagnostic Medical Sonographers (ARDMS) (www.ardms.org).

CCI awards professional certification to candidates who pass the Cardiovascular Science exam and one of these relevant registry examinations:

Registered Cardiac Sonographer (RCS)
http://www.cci-online.org/apprcs.html

Registered Vascular Specialist (RVS), for professionals working in the area of vascular technology
http://www.cci-online.org/apprvs.html

Registered Cardiovascular Invasive Specialist (RCIS), for professionals working in the area of Cardiac Catheterization
http://www.cci-online.org
/apprcis.html

Registered Cardiac Electrophysiology Specialist (RCES)
http://www.cci-online.org/apprces.html

Certified Cardiographic Technician (CCT), for professionals working in the areas of EKG, Holter monitoring and Stress testing
http://www.cci-online.org/appcct.html

The Sonography Principles and Instrumentation examination

administered by ARDMS is the first step toward registry for graduates from approved programs with work experience in echocardiographic and vascular technology. ARDMS offers three different credentials:

Registered Diagnostic Medical Sonographer (RDMS)
www.ardms.org/default.asp?ContentID=63

Registered Diagnostic Cardiac Sonographer (RDCS)
www.ardms.org/default.asp?ContentID=69

Registered Vascular Technologist (RVT)
www.ardms.org/default.asp?ContentID=71)

Most states do not require cardiovascular technologists to be licensed. In general, registry or certification credentials are voluntary and do not constitute a state license. However, two states now require sonographers to be licensed. The Society of Diagnostic Medical Sonography is working with other organizations and professionals to create the legal language for licensing.

More professional societies representing other specialties are expected to follow their example, so by the time you have completed your studies you may be required to sit for a licensing exam. Even if you are not required, many of your classmates and colleagues will voluntarily do so and it will become a competitive necessity for employment. As more employers become aware of the push toward credentialing, the more they will prefer to hire people who are certified or registered. In addition, some insurance carriers have begun to request or require that credentialed staff be present during patient procedures. This will likely become a stricter standard as the US healthcare system undergoes an overhaul.

There are no statistics, but simple observation suggests that most people working in this field have achieved two or more credentials. For instance, Maria Reyes, Director of the Non-Invasive Peripheral Vascular program at Carnegie Institute in Troy, Michigan, boasts six credentials: BS, RDCS, RVT, RMDS, RCS, and RVS!

Specializing in more than one area not only enhances your professional standing, but it greatly increases your career opportunities. For one thing, it is more cost-efficient for an employer to hire one person who can perform a variety of tasks. In addition, if you cannot get a job in your chosen area of expertise, you can look for work in one of your other specialties.

EARNINGS

HOURLY WAGES AND ANNUAL salaries are based on professional experience, geographic location, type of employer, and position (entry-level or supervisory). The level of education attained also plays a role, and CVTs with more credentials can command higher salaries because their cross training makes them a more valuable asset to the employer.

The average annual salary for all cardiovascular technologists and technicians approaches $50,000. ARDMS reports that the average sonographer's salary exceeds $60,000. Overall, earnings range from roughly $25,000 per year to more than $75,000.

Medical and surgical hospitals, which employ three out of four of the nation's CVTs, pay annual salaries of about $50,000. This is approximately the salary earned by those providing ambulatory services and outpatient care. CVTs working in physicians' offices, accounting for 15 percent of employment, earn roughly $55,000, on average. Salaries of those employed in medical and diagnostic laboratories are nearly $60,000.

Large metropolitan areas offer the best salaries because the cost of living is higher. A large number of hospitals and higher population of seniors in a particular area may also result in higher salaries because demand is greater.

Fringe benefits can be excellent and contribute substantially to the total value of the compensation package. Hospitals in particular offer generous packages, including medical, dental and vision coverage, life insurance, paid vacation and sick leave, retirement plans, continuing education opportunities.

EMPLOYMENT OUTLOOK

THE OUTLOOK FOR CAREERS IN cardiovascular technology is excellent, with employment expected to shoot up by more than 25 percent in coming years. The demand for care providers who specialize in the heart, vascular, and cerebrovascular systems will grow for a number of reasons.

The US population is aging, and older people have a higher incidence of cardiovascular ailments. The aging phenomenon is a result of the large population of Baby Boomers, the first of whom turned 60 in 2007, as well as to advances in medical science that extend longevity.

In addition, insurers and Medicaid administrators are increasingly inclined to cover noninvasive diagnostic procedures for early detection in order to reduce the need for expensive surgical procedures in the future.

The unfortunate fact is that Americans are not expected to reverse their unhealthy lifestyle habits anytime soon: salty, fatty, starchy diets, low rates of physical activity, high stress levels, and obesity will result in what could have been preventable heart disease and so-called cardiac events.

The greatest need for CVTs will be in areas with large senior populations. The US Census Bureau forecasts Florida will have the highest percentage of residents aged 65 – almost a third of all Floridians will be seniors by 2030. Other states whose senior population will top 25 percent in 2030, and which currently rank high on the list, include Maine, North Dakota, and Montana. In fact, in more than half of US states residents aged 65-plus will account for 20 percent or more of the population in 2030.

Opportunities will be most plentiful for CVTs who are certified or registered in more than one specialty.

GETTING STARTED

THE MOST IMPORTANT THING YOU can do after completing your professional education (besides finding a job) is to start studying for one or more of the certification and registry exams offered by Cardiovascular Credentialing International or the American Registry of Diagnostic Medical Sonographers. Achieving formal recognition of your competence in sonography, catheterization, electrophysiology or vascular technology may still be voluntary, but consider it mandatory!

As ARDMS notes:

Certification demonstrates your commitment to the profession

Certification establishes professional credentials above and beyond your college degree

Certification provides for greater earnings potential

Certification improves skills and knowledge by ensuring your education is up-to-date

Certification assures patients of your competency

One CVT who teaches students in an Associate of Science degree program in cardiopulmonary technology observes, "What people look for in this field are your credentials. We're not a licensed field, but there's a big move right now for everyone to obtain a registry. All employers are looking for registered technologists."

ARDMS makes practice exams, content outlines, and sample exam questions available at:

http://www.ardms.org
/default.asp?contentID=111

CCI directs students to the review materials that are advertised in its publication, *The Pulse*, with the warning that CCI does not endorse third-party preparatory courses.

As for finding your first job, your school will be your best source for career advice. Hudson Valley Community College (www.hvcc.edu/hsc/index.html), for one, which provides instruction in Echocardiography and Invasive Cardiovascular Technology, maintains a Center for Careers and Employment for students and alumni. The service includes online access to the Hudson Valley Community College Job Bank and the opportunity to meet one-on-one with a counselor for help with beginning the job search, identifying Web-based databases to find openings, writing résumés and cover letters, learning networking skills, practicing for interviews, researching companies, and even overcoming obstacles.

Careers in cardiovascular technology are extraordinarily rewarding, stimulating and challenging, and the outlook for this field could hardly be more promising. Keep your finger on the pulse, and good luck!

ORGANIZATIONS

- **Alliance of Cardiovascular Professionals**
  http://www.acp-online.org

- **American Institute of Ultrasound in Medicine**
  http://www.aium.org

- **American Registry for Diagnostic Medical Sonography**
  http://www.ardms.org

  - **American Society of Echocardiography**
    http://www.asecho.org

  - **Cardiovascular Credentialing International**
    http://www.cci-online.org

  - **Commission on Accreditation of Allied Health Education Programs**
    http://www.caahep.org

  - **Joint Review Committee on Education in Diagnostic Medical Sonography**
    http://www.jrcdms.org

  - **Society for Vascular Ultrasound**
    http://www.svunet.org

  - **Society of Diagnostic Medical Sonography**
    http://www.sdms.org

  - **Society of Invasive Cardiovascular Professionals**
    http://www.sicp.com

  - **American Heart Association**
    http://www.americanheart.org

PERIODICALS

- **Cath Lab Digest**
  www.cathlabdigest.com

- **The Pulse**
  www.cci-online.org/archives.html

- **Arteriosclerosis, Thrombosis, and Vascular Biology**
  http://atvb.ahajournals.org

- **CardioSource**
  http://www.cardiosource.com

- **Circulation**
  http://circ.ahajournals.org/

- **Journal of Invasive Cardiology**
  http://www.invasivecardiology.com

- **Journal for Vascular Ultrasound**
  www.svunet.org/JVU/index.htm

www.ingramcontent.com/pod-product-compliance
Lightning Source LLC
Chambersburg PA
CBHW070744180526
45168CB00004B/1529